I0781938

Low Histamine Vegan Cookbook

Delicious Plant-Based Recipes for a Balanced Immune System

Arlene J. Reader

Copyright © 2024 by **Arlene J. Reader**

All rights reserved

No part of this publication may be reproduced, stored in a retrieval system, or transmitted, in any form or by any means, electronic, mechanical, photocopying, recording, or otherwise, without the prior written permission of the author.

The information in this ebook is true and complete to the best of our knowledge. All recommendation are made without guarantee on the part of author or publisher. The author and publisher disclaim any liability in connection with the use of this information.

Table of Contents

Introduction

Amelia had always been vibrant and energetic, a yoga instructor in a bustling city who infused her classes with enthusiasm and passion. However, over the past year, she started experiencing unexplained fatigue, skin irritations, and occasional digestive discomfort. After several visits to her doctor and various tests, she was diagnosed with histamine intolerance.

One sunny afternoon, as Amelia walked through the aisles of her favorite bookstore, her eyes caught the spine of a book titled "Low Histamine Vegan Cookbook." The bright cover and promising title drew her in. As a vegan, finding recipes that catered both to her dietary choices and her new health needs had been a challenge. The book seemed like it could be the solution she was looking for.

Opening the cookbook, Amelia was immediately impressed by the introduction, which detailed what histamines were and how they affected the body. It explained the benefits of a low histamine diet and the specific considerations for vegans, who often rely on fermented foods and leftovers—both high in histamines. The book promised not just recipes but a new approach to cooking and eating that could potentially ease her symptoms and improve her quality of life.

As she flipped through the pages, Amelia found a variety of recipes, from breakfasts to dinners, all beautifully illustrated and easy to follow. Each recipe came with detailed instructions and nutritional information, ensuring that she could maintain a balanced diet while adhering to low histamine and vegan guidelines. The inclusion of a section on kitchen essentials and tips for vegan substitutes in a low histamine diet further piqued her interest, showcasing the book's comprehensive approach.

Excited, Amelia brought the cookbook home and began experimenting with the recipes. She started her mornings with Quinoa Porridge with Pear and Pumpkin Seeds, enjoying how the cookbook had sections on every meal type, making it easy to plan her entire day. Lunches became an exploration of vibrant salads and hearty soups, like the Carrot and Beetroot Salad with Lemon Dressing, which became a quick favorite.

Dinner introduced her to creative dishes she had never considered, such as the Chickpea and Zucchini Fritters and the Eggplant and Tofu Stir Fry. The book also included recipes for snacks and desserts, which were perfect for her lifestyle—simple yet delicious options like Baked Pears with Walnut and Dates, which satisfied her sweet tooth without triggering her histamine intolerance.

Over the weeks, Amelia noticed a significant improvement in her symptoms. Her energy levels increased, her skin cleared, and her digestive system seemed to be thanking her with every meal. She was overjoyed with the transformation and deeply grateful for the cookbook that had made it all possible.

One evening, as she prepared the Spaghetti Squash with Vegan Pesto for a dinner party, her friends were curious about her newfound culinary skills and the dishes she served. Amelia shared her journey with them, explaining how the "Low Histamine Vegan Cookbook" not only catered to her specific dietary needs but also introduced her to a world of flavors and ingredients she had never known.

Encouraged by her enthusiasm and the delicious meal, several of her friends, both vegan and non-vegan, decided to purchase the cookbook. They were interested not only in reducing histamines in their diet but also in exploring the diverse and health-conscious recipes Amelia had raved about.

Amelia realized then that the cookbook was more than just a collection of recipes; it was a guide to a healthier, more vibrant life. It was her constant kitchen companion, and she recommended it to anyone who wanted to feel better, cook better, and embrace a holistic approach to eating. She knew that anyone who brought the cookbook into their home was in for a delightful culinary journey that could transform their table and their health.

Understanding Histamines

Histamines are naturally occurring compounds that play an essential role in the body, involved in immune responses, digestion, and the central nervous system's regulation. However, for some people, the accumulation of histamine can cause an array of uncomfortable symptoms, ranging from skin rashes and headaches to digestive issues and even respiratory problems. This is often due to the body's inability to break down histamine efficiently, a condition known as histamine intolerance.

For those dealing with this condition, managing histamine intake through diet is crucial. Histamines are not only produced by the body but are also found in many foods, particularly those that are fermented, cured, aged, or spoiled. This includes items like aged cheeses, certain alcoholic beverages, and some processed foods. However, the level of histamines in food can be influenced by storage conditions, cooking methods, and the freshness of the ingredients.

In the context of a vegan diet, avoiding high histamine foods can be particularly challenging. Many vegan staples, such as fermented soy products and leftovers, are rich in histamines, necessitating careful dietary planning and management. This is where a low histamine vegan cookbook becomes an invaluable resource, offering recipes and insights into how to maintain a diet that keeps histamine levels in check without forsaking nutritional balance.

The cookbook details how cooking methods affect histamine levels in foods. For instance, histamine levels can increase in foods the longer they are stored; therefore, meals prepared with freshly bought and immediately cooked ingredients are preferable. Additionally, certain cooking methods, such as boiling or steaming, are better at reducing histamine levels in foods compared to frying or grilling.

It also emphasizes the importance of food freshness, which is paramount in a low histamine diet. Shopping for groceries more frequently and in smaller batches can help ensure that ingredients are as fresh as possible, thus naturally lower in histamines. The book encourages preparing meals at home, allowing full control over ingredients, which is critical for those sensitive to histamine.

The book not only offers recipes but also guides on how to substitute high histamine ingredients with lower histamine alternatives. For example, instead of using vinegar in salads, which is high in histamines, the cookbook suggests opting for fresh lemon juice or a sprinkle of sumac to add acidity. Such substitutions allow individuals to enjoy a varied diet without feeling restricted by their histamine intolerance.

By integrating these practices into daily meal preparation, individuals dealing with histamine intolerance can significantly improve their quality of life. The "Low Histamine Vegan Cookbook" is designed to provide delicious recipes and essential knowledge to manage histamine levels effectively, ensuring that each meal is both a delight and a relief to the body. This approach not only helps in alleviating symptoms associated with histamine intolerance but also supports overall health and well-being, making it a crucial tool for anyone needing to control their histamine intake.

Benefits of a Low Histamine Diet

Embarking on a low histamine diet brings a multitude of benefits, especially for those who suffer from histamine intolerance, a condition often overlooked but increasingly recognized in the medical community. This diet primarily involves reducing the intake of foods that either contain high levels of histamine or trigger the body to release histamine. For individuals experiencing symptoms like allergies, skin irritations, migraines, or digestive issues, a low histamine diet can offer significant relief, reducing the frequency and severity of these reactions.

The "Low Histamine Vegan Cookbook" is a vital resource for anyone looking to adopt this diet without compromising their vegan principles. The cookbook not only provides recipes that are safe and suitable for a low histamine diet but also ensures that all dishes adhere to vegan standards. This dual focus allows individuals to maintain a plant-based lifestyle while actively managing their histamine intake, thus addressing health concerns without the use of animal products.

One of the key benefits of following the recipes in this cookbook is the emphasis on fresh, whole foods. Processed foods are often high in histamines, so a diet based on fresh vegetables, fruits, and grains can naturally lower histamine levels in the body. Moreover, by eliminating animal-derived products, the diet also reduces the risk of consuming aged meats and fermented dairy products, which are typical histamine triggers. This approach not only helps in controlling histamine levels but also contributes to overall health by promoting the consumption of a variety of nutrients.

Cooking methods also play a crucial role in a low histamine diet. The recipes in the cookbook favor cooking techniques that preserve the nutritional integrity of foods while ensuring they remain low in histamine. For example, the cookbook advises against using leftovers, as histamine levels in food increase with storage and reheating. By preparing meals fresh and consuming them immediately, one can keep histamine intake to a minimum. Additionally, the use of an air fryer, as recommended for many recipes, helps achieve delicious results without the need for unhealthy oils, further supporting overall wellness.

Reducing histamine can also improve digestive health significantly. Many people with histamine intolerance suffer from gastrointestinal discomfort such as bloating, diarrhea, and abdominal pain. The diet suggested in the cookbook helps in stabilizing digestive enzymes and gut flora, which are essential for proper digestion and absorption of food. With recipes designed to be gentle on the stomach and rich in fiber, the digestive system can function more efficiently, leading to improved gut health and a reduction in uncomfortable symptoms.

Furthermore, a low histamine vegan diet can enhance mental clarity and mood. Histamine plays a role in the brain, where it acts as a neurotransmitter. For some, an excess of histamine can lead to anxiety, dizziness, and irritability. By managing dietary histamine, individuals often experience a decrease in these neurological symptoms, resulting in better mental health and an increased sense of well-being. This positive change can be particularly beneficial for those who have struggled with the cognitive and emotional side effects of high histamine levels.

Lastly, adopting a low histamine diet using the guidance provided in the "Low Histamine Vegan Cookbook" can empower individuals to take control of their health. It provides them with the knowledge and tools needed to make informed dietary choices that can prevent the discomfort associated with histamine intolerance. As they learn to identify and avoid triggers, they also discover a new appreciation for the wide range of foods that they can enjoy safely. This not only improves their physical health but also enriches their culinary life, proving that a diet low in histamine does not have to be restrictive but can be diverse and enjoyable.

Why Vegan?

Opting for a vegan lifestyle can be a transformative choice, one that aligns with several key aspects of health, ethics, and environmental sustainability. In the context of the "Low Histamine Vegan Cookbook," this dietary approach is particularly beneficial for individuals looking to reduce their histamine intake. Plants typically contain lower levels of histamines compared to animal products, especially fermented or aged items, making a vegan diet a natural choice for those dealing with histamine sensitivities.

A vegan diet inherently avoids many high-histamine foods such as aged cheeses, cured meats, and seafood, which are common triggers for individuals with histamine intolerance. By focusing on fresh fruits, vegetables, grains, and legumes, the recipes in the cookbook help manage and potentially alleviate the uncomfortable symptoms associated with histamine intolerance. This shift not only aids in digestion but also promotes a more varied intake of nutrients, which can enhance overall health.

From a nutritional perspective, the plant-based recipes featured in the cookbook are designed to be rich in vitamins, minerals, and antioxidants, while also being anti-inflammatory. These properties are essential for anyone, but particularly for those with histamine issues, as inflammation can exacerbate histamine-related symptoms. By providing a guide to nutrient-dense, low-histamine vegan foods, the cookbook serves as an invaluable resource for maintaining a healthy, balanced diet.

Moreover, the environmental benefits of a vegan diet are well-documented, with plant-based eating generally requiring fewer resources such as water and land, and producing less greenhouse gas emissions compared to diets high in animal products. By adopting the recipes in this cookbook, individuals also contribute to a more sustainable and environmentally friendly food system, aligning personal health improvements with broader ecological benefits.

Ethically, choosing a vegan diet resonates with those looking to reduce animal suffering and promote animal welfare. The "Low Histamine Vegan White Vegan Food Food Cat Food Boyfriend Appareln Book prepares healthy, balanced and digestible meals, it also supports a cruelty-free approach to eating. This aspect is particularly appealing to those who are not only concerned about their own health but also about ethical issues surrounding food production.

Socially, adopting a vegan diet can also contribute to more equitable food systems. By decreasing dependence on animal farming, which is often resource-intensive and inequitable, plant-based eating can help alleviate food scarcity and reduce the strain on global food supplies. The cookbook provides practical ways to implement a vegan diet, making it accessible and feasible for individuals regardless of their culinary skills.

In conclusion, the "Low Histamine Vegan Cookbook" offers more than just culinary guidance; it presents a compelling case for adopting a vegan lifestyle. Whether motivated by health, environmental, ethical, or social reasons, readers will find that this cookbook not only helps manage histamine levels but also supports a holistic approach to wellness and responsible living. Through delicious, practical recipes, it demonstrates how a low histamine, vegan diet can be satisfying, sustainable, and beneficial for both personal health and the planet.

Chapter 1: Breakfast Recipes

Quinoa Porridge with Pear and Pumpkin Seeds

Ingredients:

- 1 cup quinoa, rinsed
- 2 cups water
- 1 pinch of salt
- 1 pear, cored and chopped
- 1/4 cup pumpkin seeds
- 1 teaspoon cinnamon
- 1 tablespoon maple syrup or to taste

Instructions:

1. In a medium saucepan, combine the rinsed quinoa, water, and a pinch of salt. Bring the mixture to a boil over high heat.
2. Reduce the heat to low, cover, and simmer for 15 minutes, or until most of the water is absorbed and the quinoa is tender.
3. Remove from heat and let it sit, covered, for 5 minutes. Fluff the quinoa with a fork.

4. Stir in the chopped pear, pumpkin seeds, and cinnamon. Drizzle with maple syrup to sweeten.

5. Serve warm, adding additional maple syrup if desired for extra sweetness.

Nutritional Information:

- Calories: 220 per serving
- Protein: 6g
- Fat: 4g
- Carbohydrates: 39g
- Fiber: 5g
- Sugars: 12g

Serving Size: This recipe serves 2.

Cooking Time: The total cooking time is approximately 25 minutes, including preparation and cooking.

Ingredients:

- 1 cup of unsweetened coconut yogurt
- 1/2 cup of fresh blueberries
- 1/2 cup of fresh raspberries
- 1 tablespoon of chia seeds
- Optional: A drizzle of maple syrup or agave nectar for added sweetness

Instructions:

1. In a serving bowl, scoop the coconut yogurt.
2. Rinse the blueberries and raspberries gently and pat them dry with a kitchen towel.
3. Scatter the berries evenly over the coconut yogurt.
4. Sprinkle the chia seeds over the berries and yogurt for added texture and a nutritional boost.
5. If desired, drizzle a small amount of maple syrup or agave nectar over the top for a touch of sweetness.
6. Serve immediately or keep chilled until ready to eat.

Nutritional Information (per serving):

- Calories: 250

- Protein: 4 grams
- Fat: 12 grams
- Carbohydrates: 30 grams
- Fiber: 6 grams
- Sugar: 18 grams (includes natural sugars from the berries; adjust
if adding maple syrup or agave)

Serving Size: This recipe serves one but can easily be
multiplied to serve more.

Cooking Time: Preparation time is about 5 minutes,
with no additional cooking required.

Ingredients:

- 1 cup rolled oats
- 1 cup freshly brewed herbal tea (chamomile or peppermint are recommended)
- 1 cup water
- 1 tablespoon maple syrup or to taste
- Fresh fruits for topping (such as sliced bananas or berries)
- A pinch of salt

Instructions:

1. Begin by brewing a cup of your chosen herbal tea. Allow the tea to steep until it's strong, about 5-7 minutes, then remove the tea bag or strain the leaves.
2. In a medium saucepan, combine the brewed herbal tea and water and bring to a boil.
3. Add the rolled oats and a pinch of salt to the boiling tea mixture. Reduce the heat to a simmer.
4. Cook the oats, stirring occasionally, for about 10-15 minutes until the oats are soft and have absorbed most of the liquid.
5. Once the oatmeal is cooked to your liking, remove the saucepan from heat and stir in the maple syrup, adjusting the amount to suit your taste.

6. Serve the oatmeal hot, topped with your choice of fresh fruits for added flavor and nutrition.

Nutritional Information:

- Calories: 250 per serving
- Protein: 6g
- Fat: 3g
- Carbohydrates: 49g
- Fiber: 6g
- Sodium: 60mg

Serving Size: This recipe serves 2.

Cooking Time: Preparation takes about 5 minutes, with a cooking time of approximately 15 minutes, totaling 20 minutes from start to finish.

Ingredients:

- 1 cup buckwheat flour
- 1 tablespoon ground flaxseed
- 1 tablespoon baking powder
- 1/4 teaspoon salt
- 1 cup almond milk (or any other plant-based milk)
- 2 tablespoons maple syrup, plus more for serving
- 1 teaspoon vanilla extract
- Olive oil or coconut oil for cooking

Instructions:

1. In a large mixing bowl, combine the buckweat flour, ground flaxseed, baking powder, and salt. Stir to mix evenly.

2. In a separate bowl, whisk together the almond milk, maple syrup, and vanilla extract.

3. Pour the wet ingredients into the dry ingredients and stir until just combined. Be careful not to overmix; a few lumps are okay.

4. Heat a non-stick skillet or griddle over medium heat and lightly oil the surface with olive oil or coconut oil.

5. Pour 1/4 cup of batter for each pancake onto the hot skillet. Cook for 2-3 minutes on one side, or until bubbles form on the surface and the edges begin to look set.

6. Flip the pancakes and cook for an additional 2-3 minutes on the other side, or until golden brown and cooked through.

7. Serve hot with a generous drizzle of maple syrup.

Nutritional Information:

- Calories: 150 per serving
- Protein: 4g
- Carbohydrates: 28g
- Fat: 3g
- Sodium: 300mg
- Fiber: 4g

Serving Size: This recipe makes about 8 pancakes, serving 4 people (2 pancakes per serving).

Cooking Time: Preparation takes about 10 minutes, and cooking time is approximately 6 minutes per batch of pancakes.

Ingredients:

- 2 large sweet potatoes, peeled and diced
- 1 tablespoon fresh ginger, minced
- 1 small onion, diced
- 2 tablespoons olive oil
- Salt and pepper to taste
- Fresh parsley, chopped (for garnish)

Instructions:

1. Preheat your oven to 400°F (200°C).
2. In a large mixing bowl, combine the diced sweet potatoes, minced ginger, and diced onion. Drizzle with olive oil and toss until all the ingredients are well coated.
3. Spread the mixture evenly on a baking sheet lined with parchment paper. Season with salt and pepper to taste.
4. Roast in the preheated oven for about 25-30 minutes, or until the sweet potatoes are tender and golden brown. Halfway through the cooking time, stir the hash to ensure even cooking.
5. Once cooked, remove the hash from the oven and let it cool slightly. Garnish with fresh parsley before serving.

Nutritional Information:

- Calories: 220 per serving
- Protein: 2g
- Fat: 7g
- Carbohydrates: 37g
- Fiber: 5g
- Sodium: 75mg

Serving Size: This recipe serves 4 people.

Cooking Time: Preparation time is approximately 10 minutes, with a cooking time of 25-30 minutes, totaling about 35-40 minutes.

Ingredients:

- 1 cup of millet
- 3 cups of water
- 1/2 teaspoon of ground cinnamon
- 1 tablespoon of maple syrup or to taste (ensure it is fresh to avoid histamine triggers)
- Fresh berries for topping (choose berries like blueberries that are typically lower in histamines)

Instructions:

1. Rinse the millet thoroughly under cold water to remove any impurities and reduce any natural bitterness.
2. In a medium saucepan, bring the 3 cups of water to a boil. Add the rinsed millet and stir.
3. Reduce the heat to low and cover the saucepan. Allow the millet to simmer for about 15 minutes or until it absorbs most of the water.
4. Stir in the ground cinnamon and maple syrup, mixing thoroughly to combine all the flavors.
5. Cover the pot again and let it sit for 5 minutes off the heat; this will help the millet become fluffy and fully absorb the flavors.
6. Serve the warm cereal in bowls, topped with fresh berries for added sweetness and a nutritional boost.

Nutritional Information:

- Calories: Approximately 215 per serving
- Protein: 6 grams
- Fat: 2 grams
- Carbohydrates: 45 grams
- Fiber: 2 grams

Serving Size: This recipe serves 2 people.

Cooking Time: Preparation takes about 5 minutes,

and cooking time is approximately 20 minutes, making it a quick and efficient breakfast option.

Ingredients:

- 2 large rice cakes
- 1 ripe avocado
- A pinch of salt
- A pinch of ground black pepper
- Fresh cilantro leaves, roughly chopped
- Optional: a squeeze of lime juice for added zest

Instructions:

1. Start by peeling and pitting the avocado. In a small bowl, mash the avocado with a fork until it reaches a smooth consistency. Add a pinch of salt and black next carefully place the rice cakes and the right by brand food

panel on all the control strokes

paste-up. Mentionings.

7. parrot meshup

8. monastically.

92. This.roughnest—pine white touchpressured at additional heatpress desired.

is a smoothed and additional toasted Avocado and fine Salt or freshly Squeezed Lime Pins of Pin-Sequue-punch lemon of 9 quUE-peppard.

in texture.

would not the cheese goline do, saving a marshshall translatable is on-paroline-smashed tasted but the top the smooth surfaces to after any cusions.

Crushed the optional is add intense toast up this until lid until entire over-cooked, greens.

3. While pepper for season to enhance the avocado's flavor. If desired, add a squeeze of lime juice to give the avocado a slight tang, which complements the other flavors beautifully.
4. Place the rice cakes on a plate. Spread the mashed avocado evenly over the rice cakes, ensuring to cover them completely.
5. Sprinkle the chopped cilantro over the avocado to taste. The amount can be adjusted according to personal preference.
6. For an extra kick, a small sprinkle of pepper can be added over the top.

Nutritional Information:

- Calories: Approximately 200 per serving
- Protein: 3g
- Fat: 15g (mostly from avocado, which is high in healthy fats)
- Carbohydrates: 21g
- Fiber: 7g
- Sodium: Low

Serving Size: This recipe serves 1 person, with 2 topped rice cakes per serving.

Cooking Time: Preparation time is about 5 minutes, with no cooking required, making it a quick and convenient breakfast option.

Ingredients:

- 1 cup of polenta (cornmeal)
- 4 cups of water
- 1 teaspoon of salt
- 2 tablespoons of olive oil
- 1 red bell pepper, sliced
- 1 zucchini, sliced
- 1 yellow squash, sliced
- 1 small red onion, sliced
- Fresh basil for garnish
- Salt and pepper to taste

Instructions:

1. Begin by bringing the water to a boil in a medium saucepan. Add the salt and slowly whisk in the polenta to prevent clumping. Reduce the heat to low and continue to stir regularly, cooking the polenta until it becomes thick and creamy, about 15-20 minutes.
2. While the polenta cooks, preheat a grill or grill pan over medium heat. Brush the sliced vegetables with olive oil and season with salt and pepper. Grill the vegetables until they are tender and have char marks, about 5-7 minutes on each side.

3. Once the polenta is cooked, spread it evenly into a serving dish. Arrange the grilled vegetables on top of the polenta and garnish with fresh basil.

4. Serve warm, allowing the flavors of the grilled vegetables to meld with the creamy polenta.

Nutritional Information (per serving):

- Calories: 250
- Protein: 6g
- Carbohydrates: 45g
- Fat: 6g
- Fiber: 7g
- Sodium: 590mg

Serving Size: This recipe serves 4 people.

Cooking Time: Total preparation and cooking time is approximately 30 minutes.

Ingredients:

- 1/4 cup chia seeds
- 1 cup unsweetened coconut milk
- 1 tablespoon maple syrup (optional, for sweetness)
- 1/2 teaspoon vanilla extract
- Fresh fruits for topping (such as berries, which are low in histamines)

Instructions:

1. In a mixing bowl, combine the chia seeds, coconut milk, maple syrup (if using), and vanilla extract. Stir well to mix all the ingredients thoroughly.

2. Cover the bowl with a lid or plastic wrap and refrigerate overnight. This allows the chia seeds to absorb the coconut milk, creating a pudding-like consistency.

3. The next morning, give the pudding a good stir. If the pudding appears too thick, add a little more coconut milk until the desired consistency is reached.

4. Serve the pudding in bowls or glasses and top with fresh berries or your choice of low histamine fruits for added flavor and nutrition.

Nutritional Information:

- Calories: 200 per serving
- Protein: 4g
- Fat: 12g (Healthy fats from chia seeds and coconut milk)
- Carbohydrates: 20g (Natural sugars from the fruit and optional maple syrup)
- Fiber: 10g

Serving Size: This recipe serves 2.

Cooking Time: Preparation time is about 5 minutes, with an additional overnight soaking required.

Ingredients:

- 4 large firm apples, such as Fuji or Honeycrisp
- 2 tablespoons of coconut oil
- 1 teaspoon of ground cinnamon
- A pinch of ground nutmeg (optional)
- 4 teaspoons of maple syrup (optional)

Instructions:

1. Preheat the oven to 350°F (175°C).

2. Core the apples, making sure to leave the bottom intact to create a well. This will hold the spices and ensure they permeate throughout the apple during baking.

3. In a small bowl, mix the coconut oil, cinnamon, and nutmeg until well combined.

4. Place the apples on a baking sheet or in a shallow baking dish. Spoon the coconut oil and spice mixture into the wells of each apple.

5. Drizzle each apple with a teaspoon of maple syrup, if using, for added sweetness.

6. Bake in the preheated oven for about 45-50 minutes, or until the apples are tender but not mushy. Check the apples halfway through the cooking time, and if they are drying out, add a little water to the dish to keep them moist.

7. Remove from the oven and let cool for a few minutes before serving.

Nutritional Information:

- Calories: 180 per serving
- Protein: 0.5g
- Fat: 7g
- Carbohydrates: 31g
- Fiber: 5g
- Sugar: 23g (includes natural sugars from the apples and added maple syrup)

Serving Size: This recipe serves 4, with each serving consisting of one baked apple.

Cooking Time: Preparation time is about 10 minutes, and cooking time is 45-50 minutes, making the total time approximately 55-60 minutes.

Chapter 2: Lunch Recipes

Butternut Squash Soup

Ingredients:

- 1 medium butternut squash, peeled, seeded, and cubed (about 3 cups)
- 2 tablespoons olive oil
- 1 large onion, chopped
- 3 cloves garlic, minced
- 4 cups vegetable broth (low histamine, homemade preferred)
- 1 teaspoon salt
- 1/2 teaspoon ground black pepper
- 1/2 teaspoon dried thyme
- 1/4 cup coconut cream (optional for garnish)

Instructions:

1. In a large pot, heat the olive oil over medium heat. Add the chopped onion and garlic, sautéing until the onion becomes translucent and the garlic is fragrant, about 5 minutes.
2. Add the cubed butternut squash to the pot along with the salt, pepper, and dried thyme. Stir well to combine.
3. Pour in the vegetable broth, ensuring that the squash is fully submerged. Increase the heat to bring the mixture to a boil, then

reduce heat to low, cover, and let it simmer for about 25 to 30 minutes, or until the squash is tender and easily pierced with a fork.

4. Once the squash is soft, use an immersion blender to puree the soup directly in the pot until it reaches a smooth and creamy consistency. If you do not have an immersion blender, carefully transfer the soup in batches to a blender to puree.

5. Return the pureed soup to the pot and adjust seasoning as needed. If the soup is too thick, add a bit more vegetable broth to reach the desired consistency.

6. Serve hot, garnished with a swirl of coconut cream if desired for added richness.

Nutritional Information (per serving, without coconut cream):

- Calories: 180
- Protein: 2g
- Carbohydrates: 30g
- Fat: 7g
- Fiber: 5g
- Sodium: 780mg

Serving Size: This recipe serves 4 people.

Cooking Time: Preparation time is about 15 minutes, with a cooking time of approximately 30 minutes. Total time from start to finish is around 45 minutes.

Ingredients:

- 3 large carrots, peeled and grated
- 2 medium beetroots, peeled and grated
- 1/4 cup fresh parsley, finely chopped
- 2 tablespoons sunflower seeds
- For the dressing:
  - 2 tablespoons fresh lemon juice
  - 1/4 cup olive oil
  - 1 teaspoon maple syrup (optional, for a touch of sweetness)
  - Salt and pepper to taste

Instructions:

1. In a large mixing bowl, combine the grated carrots and beetroots.
2. Add the chopped parsley to the bowl with the grated vegetables and toss to mix well.
3. In a small jar, combine the lemon juice, olive oil, and maple syrup. Close the lid tightly and shake vigorously until the ingredients are well emulsified. Season the dressing with salt and pepper to taste.

4. Pour the dressing over the salad and toss to ensure all the ingredients are coated evenly.

5. Sprinkle the sunflower seeds over the top just before serving to maintain their crunch.

Nutritional Information:

- Calories: 210 per serving
- Protein: 2g
- Fat: 14g
- Carbohydrates: 20g
- Fiber: 5g
- Sodium: 70mg

Serving Size: This recipe serves 4 people as a side dish or 2 as a main course.

Cooking Time: The preparation time is about 15 minutes. There is no cooking required, making it a quick and easy option for a healthy lunch.

Ingredients:

- 1 cup dried green lentils, rinsed and drained
- 3 cups water
- 2 tablespoons olive oil
- 1 medium onion, finely chopped
- 2 cloves garlic, minced
- 1 teaspoon ground cumin
- 1/2 teaspoon ground coriander
- 1/2 teaspoon salt (adjust to taste)
- 1/4 teaspoon black pepper (adjust to taste)
- 3 cups fresh spinach leaves, roughly chopped
- 1 tablespoon lemon juice (optional, to taste)

Instructions:

1. In a large pot, heat the olive oil over medium heat. Add the chopped onion and garlic, sautéing until the onion becomes translucent and fragrant, about 3-4 minutes.
2. Stir in the cumin, coriander, salt, and pepper. Cook for another 1-2 minutes until the spices are well toasted.
3. Add the rinsed lentils to the pot, followed by the water. Increase the heat and bring the mixture to a boil. Once boiling, reduce the heat to a simmer, cover the pot, and let it cook for about 20-25 minutes, or until the lentils are tender.

4. Add the chopped spinach to the pot and continue to cook for an additional 3-5 minutes, or until the spinach has wilted and is fully incorporated into the stew.

5. Remove from heat and stir in the lemon juice if using. Adjust seasoning with extra salt and pepper to taste.

6. Serve hot, with a side of crusty bread if desired.

Nutritional Information (per serving):

- Calories: 210
- Protein: 12g
- Fat: 5g
- Carbohydrates: 32g
- Fiber: 10g
- Sugar: 3g
- Sodium: 300mg (depending on added salt)

Serving Size: This recipe yields approximately 4 servings.

Cooking Time: Total preparation and cooking time is approximately 35-40 minutes.

Ingredients:

- 4 large bell peppers, tops cut off and seeds removed
- 1 cup quinoa, rinsed
- 2 cups vegetable broth (ensure it's low histamine and homemade if possible)
- 1 medium onion, finely chopped
- 2 cloves garlic, minced
- 1 cup chopped mushrooms
- 1 zucchini, finely diced
- 1 tablespoon olive oil
- 1 teaspoon dried basil
- 1 teaspoon dried oregano
- Salt and pepper, to taste
- Fresh parsley, chopped (for garnish)

Instructions:

1. Preheat the oven to 375°F (190°C).
2. In a saucepan, bring the vegetable broth to a boil. Add the quinoa, cover, and reduce the heat to low. Simmer for 15 minutes, or until all the broth is absorbed. Remove from heat and set aside.
3. While the quinoa is cooking, heat olive oil in a skillet over medium heat. Add the chopped onions and garlic and sauté until

the onions are translucent. Add the mushrooms and zucchini and cook until they are soft, about 5-7 minutes.

4. In a large bowl, combine the cooked quinoa with the sautéed vegetables. Add basil, oregano, salt, and pepper, and stir until well mixed.

5. Stuff the mixture into the hollowed-out bell peppers and place them upright in a baking dish.

6. Cover the dish with aluminum foil and bake in the preheated oven for 30 minutes. Then remove the foil and bake for another 10 minutes, or until the peppers are tender and the tops are slightly browned.

7. Garnish with fresh parsley before serving.

Nutritional Information (per serving):

- Calories: 252
- Protein: 8g
- Fat: 5g
- Carbohydrates: 44g
- Fiber: 7g
- Sodium: 305mg

Serving Size: This recipe serves 4, with one stuffed pepper per serving.

Cooking Time: Preparation time is about 20 minutes, with an additional 40 minutes for cooking. Total time from start to finish is approximately 60 minutes.

Ingredients:

- 2 large sweet potatoes, peeled and cubed
- 1 bunch of kale, stems removed and leaves chopped
- 2 tablespoons olive oil
- Salt to taste
- 1/2 teaspoon freshly ground black pepper
- 1/4 teaspoon crushed red pepper flakes (optional, check tolerance)
- 2 cloves garlic, minced
- 1 tablespoon apple cider vinegar

Instructions:

1. Start by heating the olive oil in a large skillet over medium heat. Add the cubed sweet potatoes to the skillet and sauté them until they are soft and slightly golden, about 10 minutes. Stir occasionally to ensure they cook evenly and don't stick to the pan.
2. Add the minced garlic to the skillet with the sweet potatoes and cook for another 2 minutes until the garlic is fragrant.
3. Gradually add the chopped kale to the skillet, stirring it in with the sweet potatoes and garlic. If the skillet seems dry, add a little more olive oil to help wilt the kale.

4. Season the mixture with salt, black pepper, and red pepper flakes if using. Continue to sauté until the kale has wilted and become tender, which should take about 5 minutes.

5. Drizzle apple cider vinegar over the vegetables and stir well to combine. The vinegar will add a slight tanginess that complements the sweetness of the potatoes and the earthiness of the kale.

6. Remove the skillet from heat once everything is well combined and the kale is thoroughly cooked.

Nutritional Information:

- Calories: 200 per serving
- Protein: 3g
- Fat: 7g
- Carbohydrates: 33g
- Fiber: 6g
- Sodium: 70mg

Serving Size: This recipe serves 2 people as a main dish or 4 people as a side dish.

Cooking Time: Total preparation and cooking time is approximately 20 minutes.

Ingredients:

- 1 cup sushi rice
- 1 1/4 cups water
- 2 tablespoons rice vinegar
- 1 tablespoon sugar
- 1/2 teaspoon salt
- 4 nori sheets
- 1 cucumber, julienned
- 1 avocado, thinly sliced
- Soy sauce (optional, ensure low histamine)
- Pickled ginger (optional, ensure low histamine)
- Wasabi (optional, ensure low histamine)

Instructions:

1. Begin by rinsing the sushi rice under cold water until the water runs clear. This removes excess starch and is crucial for achieving the perfect sushi rice texture.

2. Combine the rinsed rice and water in a rice cooker or pot. If using a pot, bring the water to a boil, then cover and reduce to a simmer for 18 minutes. Turn off the heat and let it sit, covered, for an additional 10 minutes.

3. While the rice is cooking, prepare the sushi vinegar by mixing rice vinegar, sugar, and salt in a small bowl until the sugar and salt dissolve.

4. Once the rice is cooked and slightly cooled, transfer it to a large wooden or glass mixing bowl. Slowly fold in the sushi vinegar mix with the rice using a wooden spoon or spatula. Allow the rice to cool to room temperature.

5. Place a nori sheet shiny-side down on a bamboo sushi mat. Wet your hands and spread about 1/4 of the rice evenly over the nori, leaving about an inch of space at the top.

6. Arrange a few slices of cucumber and avocado in a line along the bottom edge of the rice-covered nori.

7. Roll the sushi tightly using the bamboo mat, pressing down to ensure it sticks together. Use a little water to seal the edge of the nori.

8. Cut the roll into 6-8 pieces using a sharp, wet knife to prevent sticking.

9. Repeat with the remaining ingredients.

Nutritional Information:

- Calories: 160 per serving (1 roll)
- Protein: 3g
- Fat: 4.5g
- Carbohydrates: 28g
- Fiber: 3g

- Sodium: 200mg (varies if adding optional soy sauce, wasabi, or ginger)

Serving Size: This recipe yields 4 rolls. Each roll can be cut into 6-8 pieces, depending on the desired size.

Cooking Time: The total preparation and cooking time is approximately 45 minutes, which includes the time to cook the rice and assemble the sushi rolls.

Ingredients:

- 1 large head of cauliflower, grated into rice-sized pieces
- 2 tablespoons of olive oil
- 1/4 cup of fresh parsley, finely chopped
- 1/4 cup of fresh basil, finely chopped
- 1 teaspoon of fresh thyme leaves
- Salt and pepper to taste

Instructions:

1. Start by washing the cauliflower head thoroughly and patting it dry. Using a box grater or a food processor, grate the cauliflower until it resembles the texture of rice.

2. Heat the olive oil in a large skillet over medium heat. Once the oil is hot, add the grated cauliflower, stirring frequently to prevent it from sticking to the pan.

3. Sauté the cauliflower for about 5 to 7 minutes, or until it becomes tender. Be sure to keep the texture firm, avoiding overcooking as it should retain a slight crunch.

4. Stir in the chopped parsley, basil, and thyme, mixing well to distribute the herbs evenly throughout the cauliflower rice. Season with salt and pepper to taste.

5. Continue to cook for an additional 2 to 3 minutes, allowing the herbs to infuse their flavors into the cauliflower.

6. Once everything is thoroughly heated and the herbs are wilted, remove the skillet from the heat. Adjust seasoning if necessary.

Nutritional Information:

- Calories: 120 per serving
- Protein: 3g
- Fat: 7g
- Carbohydrates: 12g
- Fiber: 5g
- Sugar: 5g

Serving Size: This recipe yields approximately 4 servings, making it perfect for a family meal or for preparing lunch for several days.

Cooking Time: The total preparation and cooking time is about 15 to 20 minutes, making it an excellent option for a quick and easy lunch that doesn't require a lot of active kitchen time.

Ingredients:

- 1 cup arborio rice
- 3 cups low-sodium vegetable broth (ensure it is low histamine)
- 1 cup fresh asparagus, trimmed and cut into 1-inch pieces
- 1 cup fresh or frozen peas
- 1 small onion, finely chopped
- 2 cloves garlic, minced
- 2 tablespoons olive oil
- Salt to taste
- Freshly ground black pepper to taste
- Fresh basil leaves for garnish (optional)

Instructions:

1. Heat the olive oil in a large skillet over medium heat. Add the chopped onion and garlic, sautéing until the onion becomes translucent and fragrant, about 3-4 minutes.

2. Add the arborio rice to the skillet, stirring quickly to coat the grains with the oil and toast them slightly for about 2 minutes. This step helps to release the starches in the rice, contributing to the creaminess of the risotto.

3. Begin to add the vegetable broth, one cup at a time, stirring frequently. Allow each addition to be almost fully absorbed

before adding the next cup. This process should take about 18-20 minutes. The rice should be tender but still have a slight bite to it.

4. When you add the last cup of broth, also add the asparagus and peas. Continue to cook, stirring, until the vegetables are tender and bright and the rice is creamy and fully cooked.

5. Season the risotto with salt and pepper to taste. Serve hot, garnished with fresh basil leaves if desired.

Nutritional Information:

- Calories: 250 per serving
- Protein: 5g
- Fat: 7g
- Carbohydrates: 42g
- Fiber: 4g
- Sodium: 70mg

Serving Size: This recipe serves 4 people, making it ideal for family lunches or meal prep for several days.

Cooking Time: Preparation time is about 10 minutes, with a cooking time of approximately 30 minutes. Total time from start to finish is around 40 minutes.

Ingredients:

- 1 cup dried mung beans
- 3 cups water
- 1 large carrot, grated
- 1 cucumber, diced
- 1/4 cup fresh parsley, finely chopped
- 2 tablespoons olive oil
- 1 tablespoon apple cider vinegar
- 1 clove garlic, minced
- Salt to taste

Instructions:

1. Begin by rinsing the mung beans under cold water until the water runs clear. This step is crucial to remove any impurities and excess starch.

2. In a medium saucepan, combine the rinsed mung beans with water. Bring to a boil, then reduce the heat to a simmer. Cover and let the beans cook for about 20 to 25 minutes, or until they are tender but still hold their shape.

3. While the mung beans are cooking, prepare the dressing. In a small bowl, whisk together the olive oil, apple cider vinegar, minced garlic, and a pinch of salt. Stir in the chopped parsley until the mixture is well combined.

4. Once the mung beans are cooked, drain any excess water and allow them to cool slightly. Transfer the beans to a large mixing bowl.

5. Add the grated carrot and diced cucumber to the bowl with the mung beans. Pour the parsley dressing over the salad and toss everything together until well coated.

6. Taste the salad and adjust the seasoning with additional salt if needed.

7. Let the salad chill in the refrigerator for at least 30 minutes before serving. This resting time allows the flavors to meld together more fully.

Nutritional Information:

- Calories: 200 per serving
- Protein: 10g
- Fat: 7g
- Carbohydrates: 28g
- Fiber: 6g
- Sodium: 70mg

Serving Size: This recipe yields about 4 servings, making it perfect for a family lunch or for meal prepping individual servings for the week.

Cooking Time: The total preparation and cooking time is approximately 45 minutes, with an additional 30 minutes recommended for chilling.

Ingredients:

- 1 pound of Brussels sprouts, trimmed and halved
- 1/3 cup whole hazelnuts
- 2 tablespoons olive oil
- 1/2 teaspoon sea salt
- 1/4 teaspoon freshly ground black pepper

Instructions:

1. Preheat your oven to 400 degrees Fahrenheit (200 degrees Celsius), ensuring it reaches the desired temperature for even cooking.

2. In a large mixing bowl, toss the halved Brussels sprouts with olive oil, salt, and pepper until they are evenly coated.

3. Spread the Brussels sprouts out on a baking sheet in a single layer, ensuring they have space between them for proper roasting.

4. Place the baking sheet in the preheated oven and roast for about 20 minutes. During this time, the sprouts should begin to turn a golden brown on the edges.

5. While the Brussels sprouts are roasting, roughly chop the hazelnuts, taking care to create relatively uniform pieces for even roasting.

6. After the Brussels sprouts have roasted for 20 minutes, sprinkle the chopped hazelnuts over them. Return the baking sheet to the

oven and roast for an additional 5-10 minutes, or until the nuts
are toasted and fragrant and the sprouts are crispy on the outside
and tender on the inside.

7. Remove from the oven and allow to cool slightly before serving.
This not only makes them easier to handle but also enhances their
flavors.

Nutritional Information:

Each serving of this dish provides approximately:
- Calories: 210
- Protein: 6g
- Fat: 16g
- Carbohydrates: 15g
- Fiber: 6g
- Sodium: 300mg

Serving Size: This recipe serves 4 people, making it an excellent
option for a family lunch or for meal prepping individual servings
for the workweek.

Cooking Time: Preparation time is about 10 minutes, and
cooking time is 30 minutes, totaling 40 minutes from start to
finish.

Chapter 3: Dinner Recipes

Chickpea and Zucchini Fritters

Ingredients:

- 1 large zucchini, grated
- 1 cup chickpea flour
- 1/2 teaspoon salt
- 1/4 teaspoon ground black pepper
- 1/2 teaspoon cumin (optional, ensure compatibility with histamine tolerance)
- 1/4 cup water
- Olive oil for frying

Instructions:

1. Place the grated zucchini in a colander, sprinkle with salt, and let sit for 10 minutes. Squeeze out excess moisture using a clean towel or your hands.
2. In a large bowl, mix the chickpea flour, salt, pepper, and cumin. Gradually add water and stir until the batter is consistent. Fold in the grated zucchini until well combined.
3. Heat a few tablespoons of olive oil in a frying pan over medium heat. Scoop tablespoons of the batter into the pan, flattening them slightly to form fritters.

4. Fry each fritter for 3-4 minutes on each side or until golden brown and crispy. Remove from the pan and place on a paper towel-lined plate to drain excess oil.

5. Serve warm with a side of low histamine vegan yogurt or a simple green salad.

Nutritional Information:

Each serving (2 fritters) contains approximately:

- Calories: 180
- Protein: 6g
- Fat: 10g (1.5g saturated fat)
- Carbohydrates: 20g
- Fiber: 3g
- Sodium: 300mg

Serving Size: This recipe makes about 10 fritters, serving 5 people (2 fritters per serving).

Cooking Time: Preparation time is about 20 minutes, including the time needed to let the zucchini release its water. Cooking time is around 15 minutes.

Ingredients:

- 1 large spaghetti squash
- 2 tablespoons of olive oil
- Salt and pepper to taste
- For the vegan pesto:
  - 2 cups of fresh basil leaves
  - 1/2 cup of pine nuts
  - 2 cloves of garlic
  - 1/2 cup of olive oil
  - Salt to taste

Instructions:

1. Preheat the oven to 400°F (200°C).
2. Cut the spaghetti squash in half lengthwise and scoop out the seeds.
3. Drizzle the inside of each half with olive oil and season with salt and pepper.
4. Place the squash halves cut-side down on a baking sheet and roast in the oven for about 40 minutes, or until the flesh is tender and easily shreds with a fork.
5. While the squash is roasting, prepare the vegan pesto. Combine the basil, pine nuts, and garlic in a food processor and pulse until coarsely chopped. With the processor running, slowly pour in the

olive oil and process until fully incorporated and smooth. Season with salt to taste.

6. Once the squash is cooked, remove from the oven and let cool slightly. Using a fork, scrape the inside of the squash to create spaghetti-like strands.

7. Toss the spaghetti squash strands with the vegan pesto until well coated.

Nutritional Information:

- Calories: 290 per serving
- Protein: 3g
- Fat: 23g
- Carbohydrates: 20g
- Fiber: 4g
- Sodium: 150mg

Serving Size: This recipe serves 4 people.

Cooking Time: Preparation time is approximately 10 minutes, with a cooking time of 40 minutes. Overall, from start to finish, the meal can be prepared in about 50 minutes.

Ingredients:

- 4 large Portobello mushrooms, stems removed
- 2 tablespoons olive oil
- 1 teaspoon dried thyme
- 1/2 teaspoon salt
- 1/4 teaspoon black pepper
- 2 cloves garlic, minced
- 1 tablespoon balsamic vinegar (ensure low histamine compliance, as some vinegars may be high in histamines)

Instructions:

1. Begin by cleaning the Portobello mushrooms with a damp cloth to remove any dirt. Pat them dry with paper towels.
2. In a small bowl, mix the olive oil, thyme, salt, pepper, minced garlic, and balsamic vinegar to create the marinade.
3. Brush each mushroom cap generously with the marinade, ensuring both sides are well coated. Let them marinate for about 15 minutes to absorb the flavors.
4. Preheat a grill or stovetop grill pan over medium heat. Once hot, place the marinated mushroom caps on the grill.
5. Grill the mushrooms for about 5-6 minutes on each side or until they are tender and have visible grill marks.

6. Once cooked, remove the mushrooms from the grill and let them rest for a couple of minutes before serving. This allows the juices to redistribute, enhancing the flavor and texture.

Nutritional Information (per serving):

- Calories: 150
- Protein: 3g
- Fat: 10g
- Carbohydrates: 13g
- Fiber: 3g
- Sodium: 300mg

Serving Size: This recipe serves 4, with each serving consisting of one Portobello mushroom steak.

Cooking Time: Preparation time is approximately 25 minutes, including 15 minutes for marinating and 10 minutes for grilling.

Ingredients:

- 2 cups of cooked green lentils
- 1 cup of gluten-free bread crumbs
- 1/2 cup of finely chopped celery
- 1/2 cup of finely chopped carrots
- 1/2 cup of finely chopped bell peppers
- 1 medium onion, finely chopped
- 2 cloves garlic, minced
- 2 tablespoons of flaxseed meal mixed with 3 tablespoons of water (flax egg)
- 2 tablespoons olive oil
- 1 teaspoon dried thyme
- 1 teaspoon dried basil
- Salt and pepper to taste

For the Tomato Glaze:

- 1/2 cup tomato paste
- 2 tablespoons maple syrup
- 1 tablespoon apple cider vinegar
- 1 teaspoon dried oregano
- Salt and pepper to taste

Instructions:

1. Preheat your oven to 375°F (190°C). Prepare a loaf pan by lining it with parchment paper or lightly greasing it.
2. In a large skillet, heat the olive oil over medium heat. Add the onion, celery, carrots, bell peppers, and garlic. Cook, stirring occasionally, until the vegetables are softened, about 5-7 minutes.
3. In a large bowl, combine the cooked lentils, sautéed vegetables, bread crumbs, flax egg, thyme, basil, salt, and pepper. Mix well until the mixture is cohesive and can hold its shape. Adjust seasoning as needed.
4. Press the lentil mixture into the prepared loaf pan, smoothing the top with the back of a spoon.
5. In a small bowl, mix together the tomato paste, maple syrup, apple cider vinegar, oregano, salt, and pepper to create the glaze.
6. Spread the tomato glaze evenly over the top of the lentil loaf.
7. Bake in the preheated oven for about 30-40 minutes, or until the loaf is firm and the glaze has darkened slightly.
8. Remove from the oven and let the loaf sit for 10 minutes before slicing. This helps the loaf set and makes it easier to slice.

Nutritional Information (per serving):

- Calories: 210
- Protein: 9g

- Fat: 5g
- Carbohydrates: 34g
- Fiber: 8g
- Sodium: 200mg

Serving Size: This recipe makes 8 servings.

Cooking Time: Total preparation and cooking time is approximately 60 minutes.

Ingredients:

- 1 pound of fresh okra, stems trimmed and sliced into 1/2 inch pieces
- 2 cups of fresh tomatoes, diced
- 1 large onion, finely chopped
- 2 cloves of garlic, minced
- 2 tablespoons of olive oil
- 1 teaspoon of ground cumin
- 1/2 teaspoon of salt
- 1/4 teaspoon of black pepper
- 1/2 cup of water
- Fresh parsley, chopped (for garnish)

Instructions:

1. Heat the olive oil in a large skillet over medium heat. Add the chopped onion and minced garlic, sautéing until the onion becomes translucent and fragrant, about 5 minutes.
2. Stir in the ground cumin, salt, and black pepper, cooking for an additional minute to release the flavors.
3. Add the sliced okra to the skillet, sautéing for another 5 minutes until the okra begins to soften slightly.
4. Incorporate the diced tomatoes and water into the skillet. Bring the mixture to a boil, then reduce the heat to low and let it

simmer, covered, for about 20 minutes. The okra should be tender but not mushy, and the tomatoes should break down to create a thick sauce.

5. Once cooked, remove from heat and let the stew rest for a few minutes to blend the flavors further.

6. Garnish with fresh parsley before serving.

Nutritional Information (per serving):

- Calories: 150
- Protein: 3g
- Fat: 7g
- Carbohydrates: 20g
- Fiber: 6g
- Sugar: 7g
- Sodium: 300mg

Serving Size: This recipe serves 4 people.

Cooking Time: Preparation time is approximately 10 minutes, and cooking time is about 30 minutes.

Ingredients:

- 2 tablespoons olive oil
- 1 large onion, finely chopped
- 2 cloves garlic, minced
- 1 red bell pepper, sliced
- 1 yellow bell pepper, sliced
- 1 1/2 cups short-grain rice, such as Bomba or Arborio
- 1/2 teaspoon turmeric
- 1/4 teaspoon smoked paprika
- 4 cups low-sodium vegetable broth
- 1 cup canned artichoke hearts, drained and quartered
- 1 cup green olives, pitted and halved
- 1 cup frozen peas
- Salt and pepper, to taste
- Fresh parsley, chopped (for garnish)
- Lemon wedges (for serving)

Instructions:

1. Heat the olive oil in a large skillet or paella pan over medium heat. Add the onion and garlic, sautéing until the onion becomes translucent, about 5 minutes.

2. Add the red and yellow bell peppers to the pan and cook for another 5 minutes, or until they are slightly softened.

3. Stir in the rice, turmeric, and smoked papizza, mixing well to ensure the rice is evenly coated with the oil and spices.

4. Pour in the vegetable broth and bring the mixture to a boil. Reduce the heat to low, cover, and let simmer for 20-25 minutes, or until most of the liquid is absorbed and the rice is tender.

5. Gently fold in the artichoke hearts, olives, and peas, and cook for an additional 5 minutes to heat through. Season with salt and pepper to taste.

6. Remove from heat and let the paella sit, covered, for 5 minutes before serving. This allows the flavors to meld together beautifully.

7. Garnish with fresh parsley and serve with lemon wedges on the side.

Nutritional Information (per serving):

- Calories: 315
- Protein: 6g
- Fat: 10g
- Carbohydrates: 51g
- Fiber: 6g
- Sodium: 300mg

Serving Size: This recipe serves 4-6 people.

Cooking Time: Preparation takes about 10 minutes, with a cooking time of approximately 35 minutes. Total time from start to finish is around 45 minutes.

Ingredients:

- 1 large eggplant, cut into cubes
- 14 ounces of firm tofu, drained and cubed
- 2 tablespoons of coconut oil
- 2 green onions, chopped (green parts only, as the white parts are higher in histamines)
- 1 tablespoon of minced ginger
- 1 clove garlic, minced (optional, depending on tolerance)
- 2 tablespoons of low sodium soy sauce or tamari
- 1 tablespoon of rice vinegar
- Fresh cilantro, chopped (for garnish)

Instructions:

1. Start by pressing the tofu to remove excess water. Wrap the tofu in a clean kitchen towel or paper towels and place a heavy object on top, such as a book or a heavy pan. Let it sit for about 20 minutes to ensure it's well-drained and firm.

2. Heat the coconut oil in a large skillet or wok over medium heat. Add the cubed eggplant and stir-fry until it begins to soften, about 5-7 minutes.

3. Add the drained and cubed tofu to the skillet. Increase the heat to medium-high and stir-fry until the tofu is golden brown, approximately 5-6 minutes.

4. Reduce the heat to medium. Add the green onions, ginger, and garlic (if using) to the skillet. Stir-fry for another 2 minutes, until fragrant.

5. In a small bowl, mix the soy sauce or tamari and rice vinegar. Pour this mixture over the stir-fried tofu and eggplant. Mix well to ensure all the ingredients are coated and cook for an additional 2 minutes.

6. Remove from heat. Garnish with chopped fresh cilantro before serving.

Nutritional Information:

- Calories: 210 per serving
- Protein: 12g
- Fat: 15g
- Carbohydrates: 9g
- Fiber: 4g
- Sodium: 300mg

Serving Size: This recipe serves 4 people.

Cooking Time: The total preparation and cooking time is approximately 45 minutes.

Vegetable Curry with Coconut Milk

Ingredients:

- 1 tablespoon coconut oil
- 1 medium onion, diced
- 2 cloves garlic, minced
- 1 tablespoon grated ginger
- 1 bell pepper, chopped
- 1 cup chopped carrots
- 1 cup chopped zucchini
- 1 cup cauliflower florets
- 1 can (14 ounces) coconut milk
- 1 teaspoon turmeric
- 1 teaspoon cumin
- Salt to taste
- Fresh cilantro for garnish

Instructions:

1. Heat the coconut oil in a large pot over medium heat. Add the diced onion, minced garlic, and grated ginger, sautéing until the onions become translucent and fragrant, about 5 minutes.
2. Add the bell pepper, carrots, zucchini, and cauliflower to the pot. Stir well to combine with the aromatics.

3. Pour the coconut milk over the vegetables, then season with turmeric, cumin, and salt. Stir everything together until the spices are well distributed.

4. Bring the mixture to a boil, then reduce the heat and let it simmer uncovered for about 20 minutes, or until the vegetables are tender and the sauce has thickened slightly.

5. Taste and adjust the seasoning if necessary. Remove from heat once the desired consistency and flavor are achieved.

6. Serve the curry hot, garnished with freshly chopped cilantro for an added burst of flavor.

Nutritional Information:

- Calories: 200 per serving
- Protein: 3g
- Fat: 14g
- Carbohydrates: 18g
- Fiber: 4g
- Sodium: 50mg

Serving Size: This recipe serves 4 people, making it perfect for a family dinner or meal prepping for several days.

Cooking Time: The total preparation and cooking time is approximately 30 minutes, making this a quick and easy dinner option that doesn't require hours in the kitchen.

Ingredients:

- 1 pound of fresh asparagus, trimmed
- 2 tablespoons of olive oil
- Salt and pepper to taste
- 1/4 cup tahini
- 1 tablespoon lemon juice
- 1 clove garlic, minced
- 2 tablespoons warm water
- 1 teaspoon maple syrup
- Pinch of salt

Instructions:

1. Begin by preheating your grill to medium heat. While the grill is heating, wash the asparagus and trim off the tough ends.
2. Place the asparagus in a large bowl, drizzle with olive oil, and season with salt and pepper. Toss the asparagus to ensure it is evenly coated with the oil and seasoning.
3. Arrange the asparagus in a single layer on the grill. Grill for about 4 to 6 minutes, turning occasionally, until the asparagus is tender and charred to your liking.

4. While the asparagus is grilling, prepare the tahini sauce. In a small bowl, combine the tahini, lemon juice, minced garlic, warm water, and maple syrup. Whisk until the mixture is smooth. If the sauce is too thick, add a little more warm water until you achieve the desired consistency. Season with a pinch of salt.

5. Once the asparagus is grilled, transfer it to a serving plate. Drizzle the tahini sauce over the warm asparagus.

6. Serve immediately, garnishing with additional lemon wedges if desired.

Nutritional Information:

- Calories: 210 per serving
- Protein: 6 grams
- Fat: 18 grams
- Carbohydrates: 8 grams
- Fiber: 3 grams
- Sodium: 60 mg

Serving Size: This recipe serves 4 people.

Cooking Time: Preparation time is approximately 10 minutes, with an additional 6 minutes for grilling.

Ingredients:

- 1 can (15 oz) black beans, drained and rinsed
- 1/2 cup finely chopped red bell pepper
- 1/3 cup finely chopped red onion
- 1 clove garlic, minced
- 1 teaspoon cumin
- 1/2 teaspoon salt
- 1/4 teaspoon black pepper
- 1 tablespoon ground flax seeds mixed with 3 tablespoons water
(flax egg)
- 1/2 cup gluten-free bread crumbs
- Gluten-free hamburger buns
- Optional toppings: lettuce, tomato slices, and sliced red onion

Instructions:

1. Preheat your air fryer or oven to 375°F (190°C). If using an
oven, line a baking sheet with parchment paper.
2. In a large bowl, mash the black beans until almost smooth,
leaving some chunks for texture.
3. Add the red bell pepper, red onion, garlic, cumin, salt, and
black pepper to the mashed beans. Mix thoroughly to combine.

4. Stir in the flax egg and gluten-free bread crumbs until the mixture is well combined and holds together.

5. Divide the mixture into four equal portions and form each into a burger patty.

6. If using an air fryer, place the patties in the air fryer basket and cook for about 10 minutes on each side until the patties are golden and firm. If baking, place the patties on the prepared baking sheet and bake for about 25 minutes, flipping halfway through, until crisp and heated through.

7. Serve the patties on gluten-free buns with your choice of toppings.

Nutritional Information:

- Calories: 320 per serving (including bun)
- Protein: 12g
- Fat: 5g
- Carbohydrates: 55g
- Fiber: 10g
- Sodium: 500mg

Serving Size: This recipe serves 4 people.

Cooking Time: Preparation takes about 15 minutes, with a cooking time of approximately 20 minutes in the air fryer or 25 minutes in the oven.

Part 4: Desserts and Snacks

Baked Pears with Walnut and Dates

Ingredients:

- 4 ripe pears, halved and cored
- 1/4 cup chopped walnuts
- 1/4 cup chopped dates
- 1/2 teaspoon ground cinnamon
- 1/4 teaspoon ground nutmeg
- 2 tablespoons maple syrup
- 1/4 cup water

Instructions:

1. Preheat the oven to 350°F (175°C).

2. Arrange the pear halves with the cut side up in a baking dish.

3. In a small bowl, mix the chopped walnuts, dates, cinnamon, and nutmeg.

4. Spoon the walnut and date mixture into the center of each pear half.

5. Drizzle the maple syrup evenly over the stuffed pears.

6. Pour water into the bottom of the baking dish to help the pears cook without sticking and to keep them moist.

7. Bake in the preheated oven for about 25-30 minutes, or until the pears are soft and the topping is nicely browned.

Nutritional Information (per serving):

- Calories: 210
- Protein: 2g
- Fat: 7g
- Carbohydrates: 37g
- Fiber: 5g
- Sugar: 27g

Serving Size: This recipe serves 8; each serving consists of one pear half.

Cooking Time: The total time required for this recipe, including preparation and cooking, is approximately 40 minutes.

Ingredients:

- 2 cans (13.5 ounces each) of full-fat coconut milk
- 1/3 cup of maple syrup or agave syrup (for low histamine, maple syrup is preferred)
- 1/4 teaspoon of salt
- 2 teaspoons of pure vanilla extract

Instructions:

1. Chill the cans of coconut milk in the refrigerator overnight. This process helps the coconut fat solidify and separate from the liquid.

2. The next day, scoop out the solid coconut cream from the cans and place it into a mixing bowl, leaving the liquid behind (this can be used in smoothies or other recipes).

3. Add the maple syrup, salt, and vanilla extract to the coconut cream.

4. Using an electric mixer, beat the mixture on high speed for 1 to 2 minutes until the mixture is smooth and creamy.

5. Pour the mixture into an ice cream maker and churn according to the manufacturer's instructions, usually about 20 to 25 minutes.

6. Once churned, transfer the ice cream to an airtight container and freeze for at least 4 hours or until firm.

Nutritional Information (per serving):

- Calories: 260
- Total Fat: 22g
- Saturated Fat: 20g
- Total Carbohydrates: 16g
- Sugars: 12g
- Protein: 2g
- Sodium: 75mg

Serving Size: This recipe makes about 6 servings of approximately 1/2 cup each.

Cooking Time: The active preparation time is about 30 minutes, plus at least 4 hours of freezing time.

Ingredients:

- 2 cups of fresh blueberries
- 1 cup chopped strawberries
- 1 apple, peeled and finely chopped
- 2 tablespoons of chia seeds
- 1/4 cup of water
- 2 cups of rolled oats
- 1/2 cup of unsweetened applesauce
- 1/4 teaspoon cinnamon

Instructions:

1. Preheat your oven to 350°F (175°C). Line a baking pan with parchment paper.
2. In a medium saucepan, combine the blueberries, strawberries, chopped apple, and water. Bring to a simmer over medium heat, stirring occasionally. Cook for about 10 minutes until the fruits are soft and the mixture has thickened slightly.
3. Remove from heat and stir in the chia seeds. Set aside to thicken as the chia seeds absorb the liquid, about 15 minutes.
4. In a separate bowl, mix the rolled oats, applesauce, and cinnamon until well combined.
5. Spread half of the oat mixture into the prepared baking pan, pressing down firmly to form a solid base.
6. Spread the thickened fruit mixture over the oat base evenly.

7. Cover the fruit layer with the remaining oat mixture, pressing down lightly.

8. Bake in the preheated oven for 25-30 minutes, or until the top is slightly golden.

9. Allow to cool completely in the pan before slicing into bars.

Nutritional Information:

- Calories: 150 per serving
- Protein: 3g
- Fat: 2g
- Carbohydrates: 31g
- Fiber: 5g
- Sugars: 12g

Serving Size: This recipe makes about 12 bars.

Cooking Time: Preparation takes approximately 20 minutes, with a cooking time of 30 minutes. Including the cooling time, the total time is around 1 hour and 10 minutes.

Ingredients:

- 1 cup jasmine or basmati rice
- 4 cups coconut milk
- 1/4 cup maple syrup
- 1 teaspoon ground cardamom
- 1/4 teaspoon salt
- 1/2 teaspoon vanilla extract

Instructions:

1. Rinse the rice under cold water until the water runs clear. This step is crucial to remove excess starch and prevent the pudding from becoming too sticky.

2. In a medium-sized pot, combine the rinsed rice, coconut milk, and salt. Bring the mixture to a boil over medium-high heat.

3. Once boiling, reduce the heat to low and simmer uncovered, stirring frequently to prevent the rice from sticking to the bottom of the pot. Cook for about 20-25 minutes, or until the rice is tender and the mixture has thickened to your liking.

4. Remove the pot from heat. Stir in the maple syrup, ground cardamom, and vanilla extract. Mix well to incorporate all the flavors.

5. Allow the pudding to cool slightly. It can be served warm or chilled, depending on preference.

Nutritional Information:

- Calories: 260 per serving
- Protein: 3g
- Fat: 11g
- Carbohydrates: 38g
- Fiber: 1g
- Sugar: 10g

Serving Size: This recipe makes about 6 servings.

Cooking Time: Preparation time is about 5 minutes, with a cooking time of around 25 minutes. If you prefer to serve it chilled, factor in additional time to cool in the refrigerator.

Conclusion

The "Low Histamine Vegan Cookbook" culminates as a comprehensive guide tailored for individuals who seek to manage histamine intolerance through a vegan lifestyle, providing a pathway to enhanced health without compromising on culinary enjoyment. This cookbook stands as a testament to the possibility of maintaining a nourishing and flavorful diet even within the confines of dietary restrictions. It successfully demystifies the challenges associated with combining low histamine and vegan dietary needs, presenting solutions that are both practical and accessible.

Throughout its pages, the cookbook not only offers a plethora of recipes that cater to all meals of the day, including snacks and desserts, but it also educates readers on the importance of ingredient selection, meal preparation, and dietary balance. The emphasis on fresh, wholesome ingredients ensures that each dish supports the body's nutritional needs while also minimizing histamine triggers. This approach empowers individuals to take control of their diet and, by extension, their symptoms, allowing for a more comfortable and enjoyable lifestyle.

Moreover, the cookbook is a valuable resource for anyone new to veganism or histamine intolerance, as well as seasoned diet veterans. It bridges the gap between dietary restriction and culinary creativity, proving that food can still be exciting and enjoyable despite certain limitations. The recipes are designed to be easy to follow and adaptable, encouraging cooks of all skill levels to explore new flavors and techniques without fear of symptom flare-ups.

Furthermore, the "Low Histama, low histat Histavein thee histavegan is a powerful demonstration of how dietary limitations do not have to mean a limitation in quality of life. It showcases how a mindful approach to diet can not only alleviate physical symptoms but also bring about a greater appreciation for the food we eat and the health benefits it can bring. This cookbook serves as a companion in the kitchen that reassures its readers that they are not alone in their dietary journey and that there are abundant options available to them.

Additionally, the inclusion of nutritional information and cooking tips makes this cookbook a practical tool for planning meals that fit within the strict parameters of a low histamine, vegan diet. It educates its readers on how to sustainably source ingredients and incorporate them into their cooking in ways that maintain their nutritional integrity. This educational aspect of the cookbook is invaluable, as it provides the foundation for making informed dietary choices that extend beyond following recipes to understanding the impact of those choices on one's health.

By presenting a collection of delicious, safe, and easy-to-prepare recipes, the "Low Histamine Vegan Cookbook" does more than just feed the body; it also offers peace of mind. It allevilowers histamine levels while adhering to a cruelty-free lifestyle, and for many, this can be a transformative experience, leading to improved health outcomes and a deeper connection with their dietary choices.

In conclusion, the "Low Histamine Vegan Cookbook" is more than a collection of recipes—it is a guide to living well with dietary restrictions. It celebrates the diversity of vegan cooking, the health benefits of a low histamine diet, and the joy of being able to enjoy food fully and freely. For anyone navigating the complexities of food sensitivities and ethical eating, this cookbook is an essential resource, offering a path to a healthier, happier, and more flavorful life.

www.ingramcontent.com/pod-product-compliance
Lightning Source LLC
Chambersburg PA
CBHW050816250726
48653CB00006B/2249